YEAST INFECTION CURE

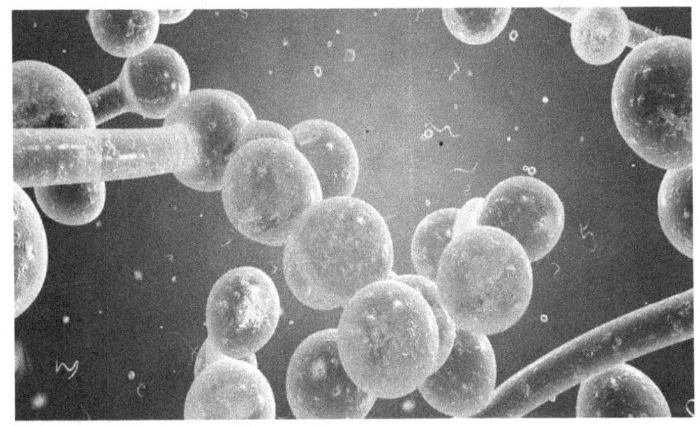

A SIMPLIFIED GUIDEBOOK TO UNDERSTANDING, DIAGNOSIS, TREATMENT, AND PREVENTION OF RECURRENT VAGINAL CANDIDIASIS IN WOMEN OF ALL AGES

DR. JOHN TAYLOR

COPYRIGHT© 2024 DR. JOHN TAYLOR

All rights reserved.

TABLE OF CONTENT

INTRODUCTION

Three out of every four A vaginal yeast infection is one of the few illnesses that affect women's health and interfere with day-to-day activities and intimate relationships. From personal relationships to work productivity, the discomfort, itching, and irritation it causes can be emotionally and physically challenging. Despite all of the discomfort and frustration, it has a very good prognosis.

Thank you for visiting "Yeast Infection Cure: a simplified guide for understanding, diagnosing, treating, and preventing vaginal candidiasis." Within these pages, you will set out on a path to understanding the causes, risk factors, signs and symptoms, prevention, and self-management of vaginal yeast infection with over-the-counter medications. Free prescriptions are provided at the end of this book to be used to get your drugs for treatment.

You would wonder, then, why a guidebook? After all, there are a ton of tips and treatments for vaginal yeast infections on the internet, right? Information is abundant, it's true, but sorting through the deluge of contradictory advice and unverified claims may be daunting and even dangerous. This guide's dedication to accuracy, clinical data, and firsthand experiences is what makes it unique.

Here, you won't find questionable "miracle cures." Instead, you'll discover a comprehensive approach rooted in clinical experience, scientific understanding, and practical wisdom. From understanding the causes and symptoms of vaginal yeast infections to exploring evidence-based treatment options and preventative strategies, each page is meticulously crafted to equip you with the knowledge and tools you need to regain control over your vaginal health.

So, whether you're experiencing your first encounter with a vaginal yeast infection or you've been battling recurrent episodes for years, know that you're not alone, and this book set you free. By embarking on this journey together, you will embrace a life free from the burdens of vaginal yeast infections.

Are you ready to unlock relief and embark on a path toward optimal vaginal health? If so, turn the

page, and let's begin. Your journey to freedom starts now.

CHAPTER 1

DEFINITION AND TYPES OF CANDIDIASIS

Overview of Candidiasis

Candidiasis is a fungal infection caused by the overgrowth of Candida species, commonly Candida albicans, which naturally inhabit various parts of the human body, including the skin, mouth, throat, gut, and genital tract. Though candida usually lives in modest quantities and gets along well with other bacteria in the body without causing any adverse outcomes, a few things can throw this equilibrium off, which can result in candidiasis.

Types of Candidiasis

Any part of the body where candida albicans exist can suffer candidiasis when the equilibrium is destabilized. Candidiasis is therefore categorized depending on the site of infection. This book is written for vaginal yeast infections.

Vaginal Yeast Infection (Vulvovaginal Candidiasis)

Vaginal yeast infection is a common type of candidiasis that affects women, particularly those of reproductive age. It is a type of reproductive tract infection but not a sexually transmitted infection because one does not have to be involved in sexual activity to get it. It occurs when there is an overgrowth of Candida in the vagina, leading to symptoms such as itching, burning, redness, swelling, and abnormal vaginal discharge (white, thick, and cottage cheese-like).

Vaginal yeast infections are often triggered by factors such as hormonal changes (e.g., pregnancy, menstruation), antibiotic use, diabetes, weakened immune system, and poor hygiene.

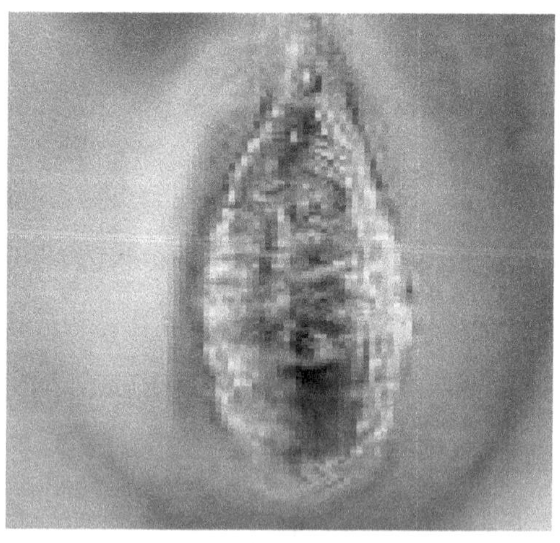

Vaginal candidiasis/yeast infection

Oral thrush is a common type of candidiasis that affects the upper gastrointestinal tract such as the mouth and throat. In the month, it presents as white, creamy patches or plaques on the tongue, inner cheeks, palate, throat, and tonsils. Oral thrush can cause discomfort, pain, burning sensation, and difficulty swallowing, especially in severe cases where it affects the throat.

Risk factors for oral thrush include a weakened immune system, HIV/AIDS, diabetes, denture use, antibiotic use, smoking, and poor oral hygiene.

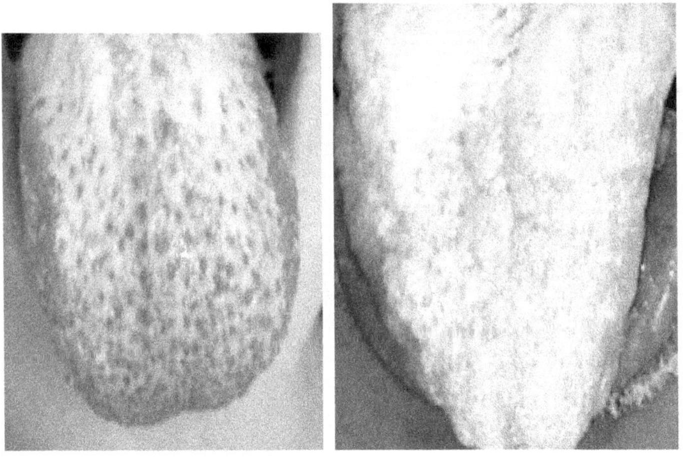

Oral candidiasis on the tongue

Cutaneous candidiasis refers to a yeast infection of the skin and nails. It typically affects warm and moist areas of the body, such as skin folds (e.g., groin, armpits), under the breasts, and between the toes. Symptoms of cutaneous candidiasis include red, inflamed patches of skin, itching, burning, and peeling.

Risk factors for cutaneous candidiasis include obesity, diabetes, excessive sweating, tight clothing, poor hygiene, and the use of occlusive dressings or topical corticosteroids.

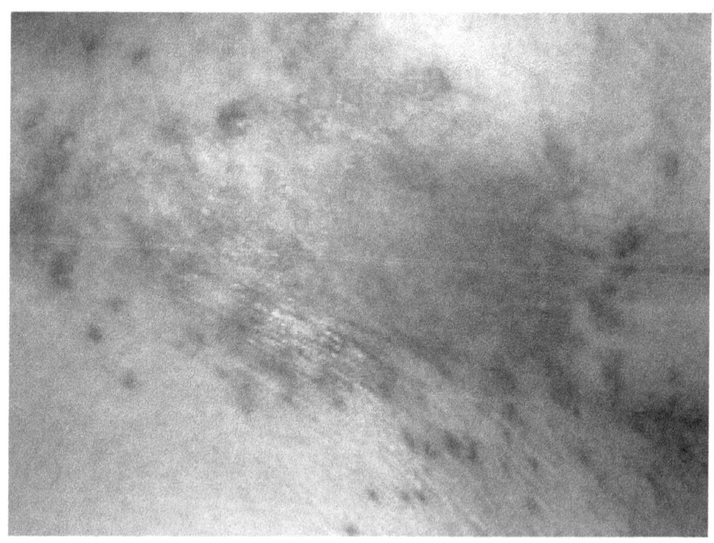

Candidiasis on the skin (under the breast)

Invasive candidiasis occurs when Candida enters the bloodstream or internal organs, leading to systemic infection. This type of candidiasis is rare but can be life-threatening, particularly in immunocompromised individuals, hospitalized patients, and those undergoing invasive medical procedures.

Symptoms of invasive candidiasis may include fever, chills, hypotension, organ dysfunction, and signs of sepsis. Invasive candidiasis requires prompt diagnosis and aggressive treatment with intravenous antifungal medications.

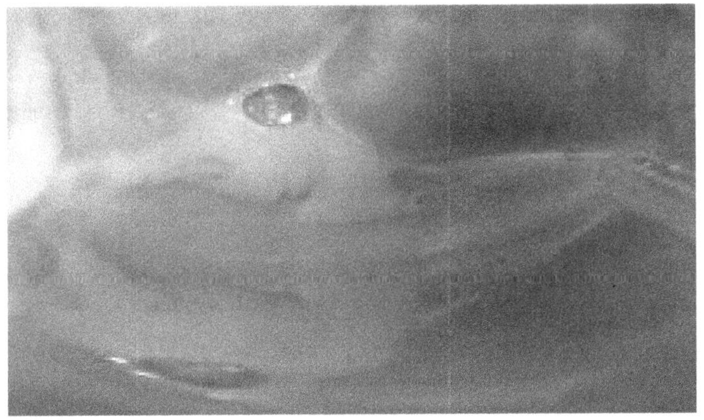

Candidiasis in the gut

Esophageal candidiasis is a type of candidiasis that affects the esophagus, the tube that connects the throat from the mouth to the stomach. It commonly occurs in individuals with weakened immune systems, such as those with HIV/AIDS, cancer, or undergoing immunosuppressive therapy. It is however possible to have esophageal candidiasis without any of these underlying medical conditions. Symptoms of esophageal candidiasis may include difficulty swallowing (dysphagia), chest pain, and odynophagia (painful swallowing). Diagnosis is typically confirmed through endoscopy and biopsy, and treatment involves antifungal therapy.

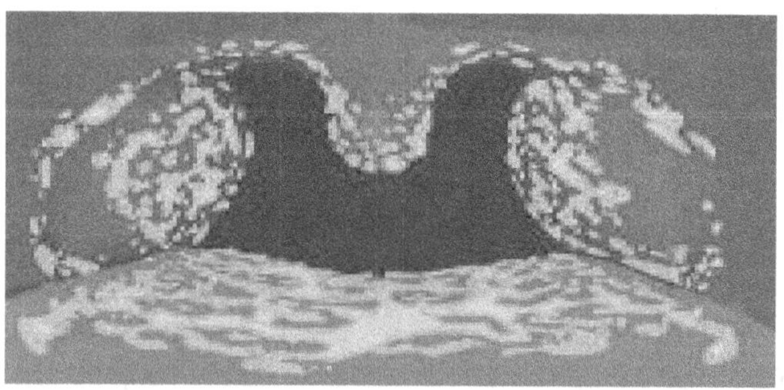

Oropharyngeal candidiasis

CHAPTER 2

CANDIDA AND RISK FACTORS

Candida Species in the Body

The vulva, vagina, and groin area may be affected by vulvovaginal candidiasis, which can be acute, chronic, recurring, or persistent. Candida affects animals and nearly all humans. One-tenth of women in their fertility ages are opportunistic carriers of the organism.

Some Candida species, including C. glabrata, C. tropicalis, and C. krusei, occur more frequently. These additional Candida species are thought to have emerged as a result of long-term suppressive drugs such as azoles, frequent short courses of antifungal medication, and self-medication

Candida Overgrowth and Vaginal Imbalance

The healthy vaginal flora of a woman during her fertility years is home to a wide variety of microorganisms. These can include both anaerobic and aerobic gram-positive and gram-negative bacteria. Other bacteria such as Streptococcus, Bacteroides, and Staphylococcus, are less common in the vagina as compared to Lactobacillus and Corynebacterium.

The production of lactic and acetic acid from glycogen by Lactobacillus and Corynebacterium helps to maintain the pH of the vagina at a lower level. These good bacteria keep other harmful bacteria in check as they are rarely harmful. If however, the environmental balance is upset, they can turn harmful.

Factors that can interfere with vaginal PH and make cause harm to the vagina include age, stage of the menstrual cycle, sexual activity, choice of contraceptive method, pregnancy, presence of necrotic tissue or foreign bodies, or the use of hygiene products or antibiotics

Candida vulvovaginitis can begin as a result of any host factor that influences the vaginal environment or secretions. A favorable habitat for Candida species is created by high levels of reproductive hormones and an increase in the glycogen content of the vaginal environment. This provides an ample source of carbon for candida germination and development.

A low vaginal pH value of less than 6 is ideal for the formation of the germ tube and the growth of mycelia, even though the organism's first attachment happens more easily at high pH values between 6 and 7.

Even though candida may be isolated in semen or vaginal secretions, it is not transmitted sexually transmitted, and sexual partners are normally not treated for candidiasis. This is because it affects celibate women too and is found to be a normal component of the vaginal flora.

Causes Vaginal Yeast infection

This handbook emphasized vaginal candidiasis also called vaginal yeast infection or vulvovaginal candidiasis. Vaginal candidiasis, as explained earlier, is a common fungal infection caused by an overgrowth of Candida species, typically Candida albicans, in the vaginal area. Other candida species that can cause candidiasis include candida glabrata, candida tropocalis, and candida krusei. These are all considered an opportunistic infection because of their habitual presence in the vaginal without causing harm until there is an imbalance in the normal vaginal flora.

Several factors increase the risk of developing yeast infection of the vagina. I have provided an elaborate explanation of the various risk factors that predispose to candidiasis. Since the organism that causes candidiasis is ever present in the vagina and body your ability to take control of them will limit its occurrence. 3 out of every 4 women experience the condition at least once in their lifetime and 2 out of 4 will experience re-occurrence. Know these risk factors and practice them to avoid the disease and its depleting effect on your life.

Douching

Douching, or the practice of rinsing or cleaning the vaginal area with water or other fluids, can disrupt the natural balance of vaginal microorganisms and increase the risk of vaginal candidiasis. Douching is generally not recommended as it can irritate the vaginal tissues and promote infections. The initial intervention by most adolescent girls when to see discharge is to wash it with water and detergent. This worsens the situation for them within a few days with severe vaginal and vulva itching and irritations.

Antibiotic Misuse

This is often encountered in medical practice. Antibiotics can disrupt the natural balance of microorganisms in the body, including the vagina, by killing beneficial bacteria that help keep Candida in check. This is particularly worse for individuals taking broad-spectrum antibiotics for systemic infections. These drugs kill the targeted organisms including beneficial bacteria in the skin, vagina, and other parts of the body, creating room for harmful organisms to flourish. This disruption can lead to an overgrowth of Candida and increase the risk of vaginal yeast infections.

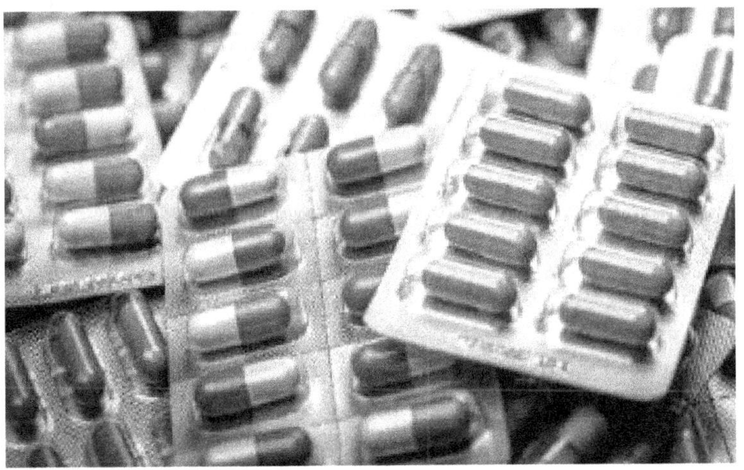

Tight or Non-Breathable Clothing

Wearing tight-fitting or non-breathable clothing, such as synthetic underwear or pantyhose, can create an environment that favors Candida growth.

Tight underwear can trap heat and moisture around the genital area, creating a warm and humid environment. This environment provides an ideal breeding ground for yeast, particularly Candida species, to overgrow and cause an infection. Yeast thrives in moist environments, and the lack of airflow caused by tight clothing can exacerbate this.

It restricts airflow to the genital area, reducing ventilation and hindering the evaporation of sweat and moisture. Adequate ventilation is essential for maintaining dryness and preventing the accumulation of moisture, which can promote yeast growth. Without proper airflow, the genital area may remain damp, facilitating the growth of Candida.

Personal Hygiene Practices

Poor personal hygiene practices, such as wearing damp or sweaty clothing for prolonged periods, using scented hygiene products (e.g., soaps, douches, sprays), or not changing tampons or pads frequently enough, can contribute to vaginal candidiasis by creating conditions conducive to yeast overgrowth.

Sexual Activity

While vaginal candidiasis is not considered a sexually transmitted infection (STI), risky sexual activity can disrupt vaginal pH and introduce bacteria or fungi into the vaginal area, potentially increasing the risk of yeast infections, particularly in women with a history of recurrent infections.

Intercourse can sometimes cause friction or microtrauma to the vaginal tissues, especially if adequate lubrication is not achieved before vaginal penetration. Sexual intercourse with objects or sex toys is also in ascendency with the majority of people inserting unclean substances such as cucumbers, bananas, and carrots in the vagina to achieve vaginal orgasm whilst causing trauma to the vagina. These traumas can create small tears or abrasions in the vaginal mucosa, which may provide entry points for Candida and other bacteria to infect the tissue and cause a yeast infection.

The use of unclean or infected objects in the vagina can also lead to the introduction of infections into the vagina. Any kind of infection affects sexual activity and pleasure. This may affect intimate relationships, social interaction, and emotional health

Sexual activity can also temporarily alter the pH of the vagina due to the introduction of semen, which is alkaline. This change in pH can create an environment that is more conducive to the growth of Candida species, leading to an increased risk of yeast infection.

Uncontrolled Diabetes Mellitus

Uncontrolled diabetes, characterized by high blood sugar levels, can provide a conducive environment for Candida species to survive and thrive. Elevated glucose levels in vaginal secretions can promote yeast growth and increase the risk of vaginal yeast infections.

Hormonal Changes

Hormonal changes, especially those brought on by pregnancy, contraceptives, menstruation, or menopause, might create a vaginal environment that is favorable to Candida overgrowth. Pregnant women are more susceptible to vaginal candidiasis due to changes in hormone levels, which can also affect vaginal pH, glycogen levels, and immunological function.

Birth control pills, patches, and hormonal intrauterine devices (IUDs) are examples of hormonal contraceptive methods that might change hormone levels and vaginal pH, which may put some women at risk for vaginal candidiasis.

Women who are pregnant may also be more susceptible to vaginal yeast infections due to hormonal changes, elevated vaginal glycogen levels, and altered immune system function. Pregnancy increases the likelihood of vaginal candidiasis, especially in the second and third trimesters.

Weakened Immune System

Individuals with weakened immune systems due to conditions such as HIV/AIDS, cancer, diabetes, and autoimmune disorders can make them more susceptible to vaginal candidiasis. Most these people also present with other forms of candidiasis such as oral thrush, oropharyngeal and cutaneous candidiasis.

Vaginal douching involves rinsing the vagina with a solution typically made of water and vinegar, baking soda, iodine, or commercial preparations. Douching is generally not recommended since it might upset the natural balance of bacteria and yeast in the vagina, which can result in some issues, including vaginal candidiasis. Some people have false beliefs that douching keeps the vagina clean and fresh but it is the opposite.

In clinical practice, ladies who have big buttocks mostly complain of vaginal discharges with normal laboratory test tests results. These ladies have the propensity to try to wash out these discharges with douching chemicals which in the long term expose them to infections. This in my opinion could be due retention of a lot of heat within the perineal area. Secondly overweight may is as a result of excess body fat which lead to increased level of glucose in the vaginal area, creating a conducive environment to yeast overgrowth

The precise mix of bacteria and yeast that live in the vagina preserves its acidic pH and inhibits the growth of potentially dangerous germs. Douching has the potential to upset this equilibrium by eliminating the helpful bacteria that regulate yeast numbers. Due to this disruption, yeast especially Candida species can flourish and proliferate uncontrollably.

The acidity of the vagina, which is maintained by beneficial bacteria, helps inhibit the growth of Candida species. However, douching can raise the vaginal pH, making it less acidic and more hospitable to yeast overgrowth. This shift in pH creates favorable conditions for Candida to flourish.

The vagina produces a natural mucus that acts as a protective barrier against pathogens, including yeast. Douching can wash away this protective mucus layer, leaving the vaginal tissues more vulnerable to colonization by Candida species.

Some of the substances used in douching solutions, such as harsh chemicals or fragrances, can as well irritate the delicate tissues of the vagina. Irritation can disrupt the vaginal epithelium, creating microtears or inflammation that provide entry points for Candida to infect the tissue.

Even though it sometimes temporarily alleviates symptoms of vaginal infections like odor or discharge, it doesn't address the underlying cause of the infection and may rather exacerbate it.

In short, while vaginal douching may seem like a quick fix for vaginal discomfort such as discharge and itching, it's generally unnecessary and can do more harm than good. Maintaining good vaginal health typically involves gentle cleansing with water and mild, unscented soap on the external genitalia, along with practicing safe sex and avoiding unnecessary interventions that disrupt the natural balance of the vaginal ecosystem.

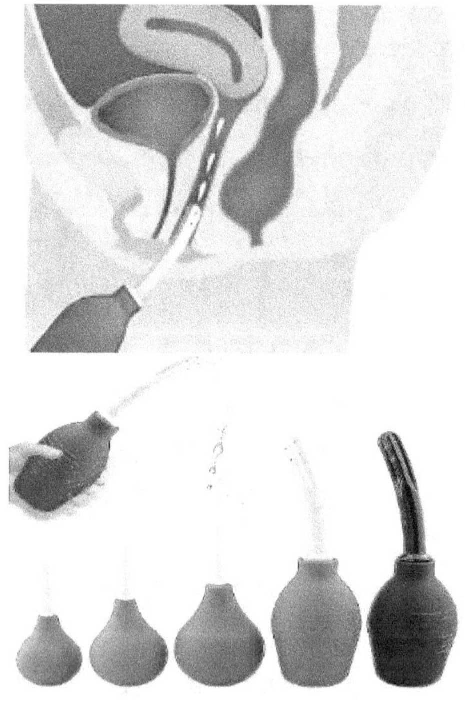

Vaginal douching and douching products

CHAPTER 3

DIAGNOSING VULVOVAGINAL INFECTIONS

Common Symptoms of Vaginal Yeast Infection

Differentiating vaginal candidiasis (yeast infection) symptoms from those of other vaginal infections can be challenging as many infections share similar symptoms. However, certain characteristics may help distinguish vaginal candidiasis from other types of vaginal infections. Even though vaginal infections are numerous, the most common vaginal infections include vaginal candidiasis, trichomoniasis, and bacterial vaginosis. Clinicians sometimes treat these infections together due to their co-existence but it is important to be able to identify the dominant infection and target treatment to it.

Vulvovaginitis is a term used to refer to any infections affecting the vagina and the vulva. Some of these other infections include atrophic vaginitis, genital herpes, cervicitis, and sexually transmitted infections such as gonorrhea and chlamydia.

Differentiating reproductive tract infections from other infections is therefore dependent on your clinical knowledge of the signs and symptoms of the various diseases. Some infections may be acquired through the reproductive tract but their effect is systemic whilst others are localized to the vagina, vulva, and cervix.

Differences Between Vaginal Candidiasis and Other Vaginal Infections

Symptoms/ diseases	Vaginal candidiasis	Trichomoniasis	Bacterial vaginosis
Vaginal discharge	thick, white, and cottage cheese-like	frothy, greenish-yellow, or grayish-white in color. Foul smelling odor	thin, watery, grayish-white or yellowish color and fishy odor
Vulva itching	Common, intense and persistent	Itchy	Mild itching
Burning sensation	During sex and urination	burning, and irritation	Not significant
Redness and swelling	red, swollen, and irritated	can cause redness, swelling	Not significant

Vaginal discharge

This is the most common symptom presented with vaginal infections. The discharge in vaginal candidiasis is typically thick, white, and cottage cheese-like in consistency. Unlike bacterial vaginosis (BV) and trichomoniasis, vaginal candidiasis typically does not cause a strong or foul odor.

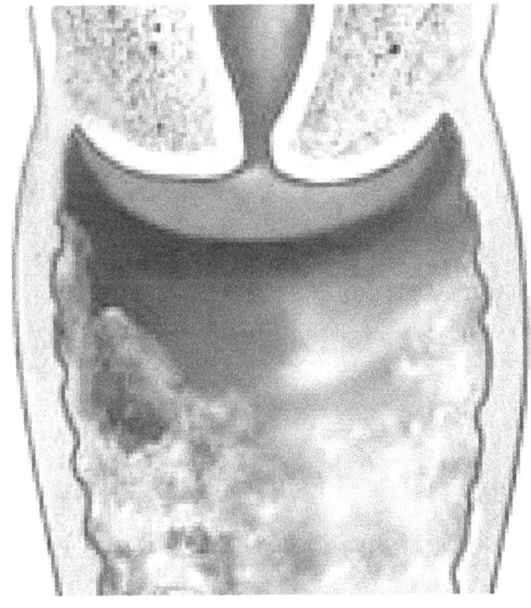

Discharge in Vaginal Candidiasis

Vulva Itching

Vaginal itching is a common symptom of vaginal candidiasis, often described as intense and persistent. Most people with vaginal candidiasis or yeast infections complain about vulva or vaginal itching.

Redness and Swelling

The vulva (outer genital area) may appear red, swollen, and irritated in vaginal candidiasis. This can also be worsened by intense scratching due to itching the vulva.

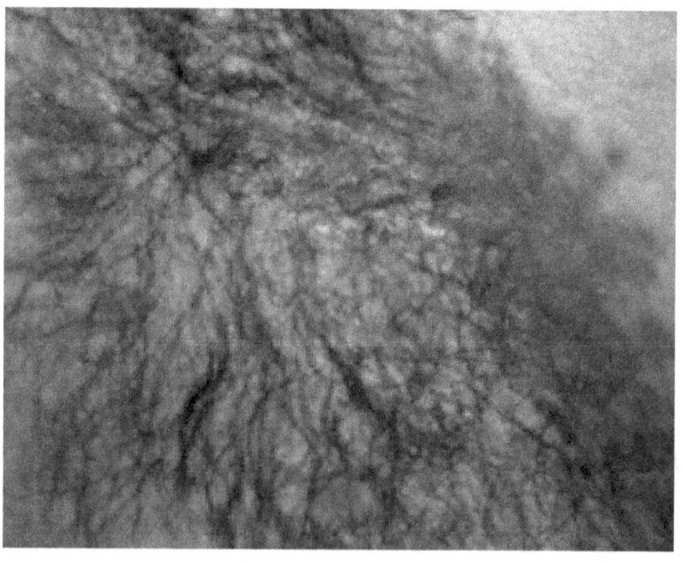

Redness and swelling in yeast infection

Burning Sensation

Some individuals with vaginal candidiasis experience a burning sensation, particularly during urination or sexual intercourse. This is normally due to intense itching leading to scratching and subsequently bruises. When drops of urine touch this bruise during urination, it burns and irritates. Prompt treatment to prevent scratching and subsequently bruises and other infections is highly recommended

Symptoms of Bacterial Vaginosis (BV)

Vaginal Discharge

The discharge in BV is usually thin, watery, and grayish-white or yellowish in color. It is normally characterized by a strong, fishy odor that becomes more noticeable after sexual intercourse or during menstruation.

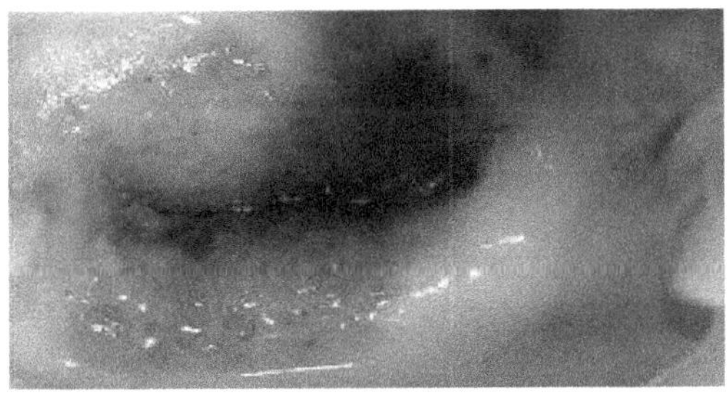

Vaginal Discharge in Trichomoniasis

Itching or Burning

Some individuals with BV may experience mild itching or burning, but it is less common compared to vaginal candidiasis.

No Significant Redness or Swelling

Bacterial vaginosis does not typically cause significant redness, swelling, or vulva irritation.

Symptoms of Trichomoniasis

Vaginal Discharge

The discharge in trichomoniasis is typically frothy, greenish-yellow, or grayish-white in color. Trichomoniasis is associated with a strong, unpleasant odor, often described as "rotten" "foul-smelling" or "phlegmy."

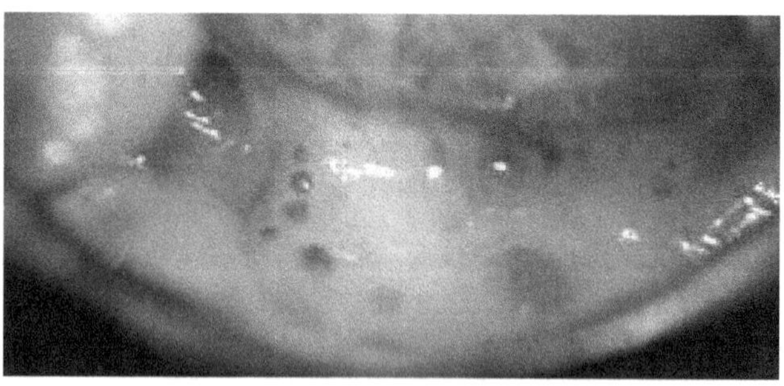

Discharge in Bacterial Vaginosis

Itching and Burning

Itching, burning, and irritation of the vagina and vulva are also a common symptom of trichomoniasis.

Redness and Swelling

Trichomoniasis can cause redness, swelling, and inflammation of the vulva and vaginal tissues but is not a common symptom.

Symptoms of Other Vaginal Infections

Other vaginal infections, such as yeast infections caused by non-Candida species, may present with similar symptoms to vaginal candidiasis. Additionally, conditions such as dermatitis, allergic reactions, genital herpes, and sexually transmitted infections (STIs) may cause symptoms similar to those of vaginal candidiasis.

Overall, while there may be overlap in symptoms among different vaginal infections, the characteristics of the vaginal discharge, presence or absence of odor, and accompanying symptoms such as itching, burning, and redness can help differentiate vaginal candidiasis from other types of infections.

Examination findings in vaginal candidiasis typically involve visual inspection of the external genitalia (vulva) and internal examination of the vagina. Here are the common examination findings associated with vaginal candidiasis:

Vulvar Redness and Swelling

The vulva, which includes the labia majora, labia minora, clitoris, and vaginal opening, may appear red, inflamed, and swollen in cases of vaginal candidiasis. Redness and swelling are signs of irritation and inflammation caused by the overgrowth of Candida fungi in the vaginal area.

Vaginal Discharge

The vaginal discharge in candidiasis is typically thick, white, and cottage cheese-like in consistency. The discharge may adhere to the vaginal walls and may be observed during the examination.

Vaginal Wall Inflammation (Vaginitis)

The vaginal walls may appear red, irritated, and inflamed during a speculum examination. Inflammation of the vaginal mucosa is a common finding in vaginal candidiasis and contributes to symptoms such as itching and discomfort.

Vaginal Discharge pH

The pH of the vaginal discharge may be tested using a pH strip during the examination. Vaginal candidiasis typically results in a normal to slightly elevated vaginal pH (pH > 4.5), distinguishing it from conditions such as bacterial vaginosis

Presence of Vaginal Candida Hyphae or Spores

Microscopic examination of vaginal secretions may reveal the presence of Candida hyphae (elongated fungal structures) or yeast cells. A saline or potassium hydroxide (KOH) wet mount preparation of vaginal discharge may be performed to visualize Candida organisms under a microscope.

Absence of Odor

Unlike bacterial vaginosis (BV), which is associated with a characteristic "fishy" odor, vaginal candidiasis typically does not cause a significant odor. The absence of a foul odor is another distinguishing feature of vaginal candidiasis during examination.

If examination findings are suggestive of vaginal candidiasis, a definitive diagnosis still requires laboratory confirmation through microscopy or culture of vaginal specimens.

Additionally, consider other factors such as clinical symptoms, medical history, and risk factors when diagnosing and managing vaginal candidiasis. For instance, the social history of multiple sexual partners may warrant evaluation for sexually transmitted diseases such as gonorrhea, syphilis, and chlamydia. Other accompanying symptoms will give a clue of urinary tract infections or other pelvic inflammatory diseases.

Differential Diagnosis

When evaluating a patient with symptoms suggestive of vaginal candidiasis, healthcare providers consider a differential diagnosis to rule out other possible causes of vaginal symptoms. The following are some common conditions that may be considered in the differential diagnosis of vaginal candidiasis:

Bacterial Vaginosis (BV)

Bacterial vaginosis is a common vaginal infection caused by an imbalance of bacteria in the vagina, resulting in symptoms such as a thin, grayish-white vaginal discharge with a characteristic fishy odor. BV is differentiated from candidiasis based on the type of discharge (thin and fishy-smelling), vaginal pH (elevated), and microscopic examination (presence of clue cells).

Trichomoniasis

Trichomoniasis is caused by the parasite Trichomonas vaginalis and is considered a sexually transmitted infection (STI). It can present with symptoms such as frothy, greenish-yellow vaginal discharge, vaginal itching, and vulvar irritation.

Trichomoniasis is diagnosed through laboratory testing, including wet mount microscopy or nucleic acid amplification tests (NAATs).

Atrophic Vaginitis

Atrophic vaginitis is inflammation of the vaginal tissues due to decreased estrogen levels, commonly occurring in menopausal women. Symptoms may include vaginal dryness, itching, burning, and dyspareunia (painful intercourse). Unlike candidiasis, atrophic vaginitis is not associated with abnormal vaginal discharge, and the vaginal pH may be elevated.

Contact Dermatitis

Contact dermatitis of the vulva and vagina can result from exposure to irritants or allergens present in personal hygiene products, detergents, soaps, perfumes, or latex condoms. Signs and symptoms mostly include itching, burning sensation, redness, and swelling.

Unlike candidiasis, contact dermatitis is typically not associated with vaginal discharge or vaginal pH changes.

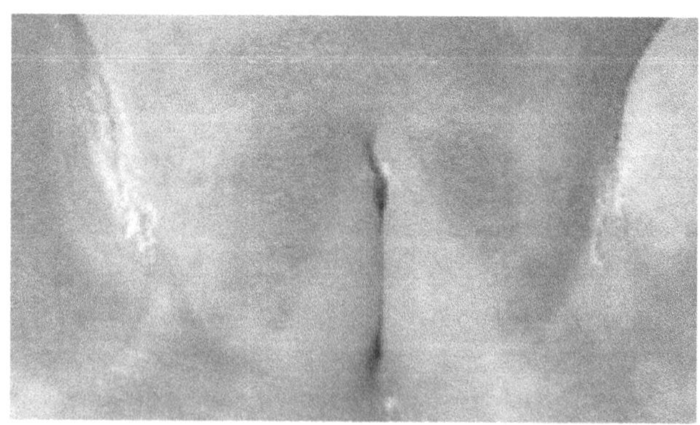

Allergic Contact Dermatitis

Genital Herpes

Genital herpes is a viral disease that is transmitted by sexual intercourse. The virus responsible is the herpes simplex virus (HSV). Symptoms mimic other vaginal infections and may include painful lesions on the genitals, vulva itching, burning sensation, and flu-like symptoms such as fever and malaise

While vaginal candidiasis does not typically cause genital lesions, genital herpes may present with vesicular or ulcerative lesions on the vulva, vagina, or perineum.

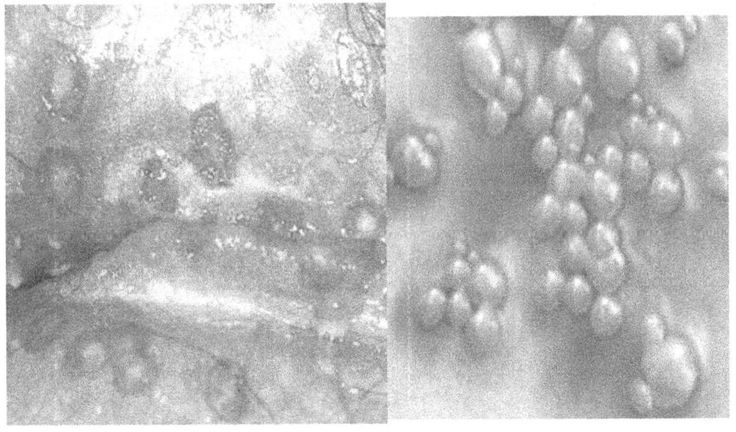

Signs of genital herpes

Gonorrhea and Chlamydia

Gonorrhea, chlamydia, and syphilis are common bacterial STIs that can infect the genital tract, including the vagina.

Symptoms may include abnormal vaginal discharge, vaginal itching, pelvic pain, dysuria (painful urination), and bleeding between periods. Laboratory testing, such as NAATs, is used to diagnose gonorrhea and chlamydia.

Yeast Infection in Men-Balanitis

Yeast infection in men is known as balanitis and presents with itching and dermatitis of the penis. It is rare in men but in situations where it occurs in men, the treatment is oral fluconazole or clotrimazole depending on severity

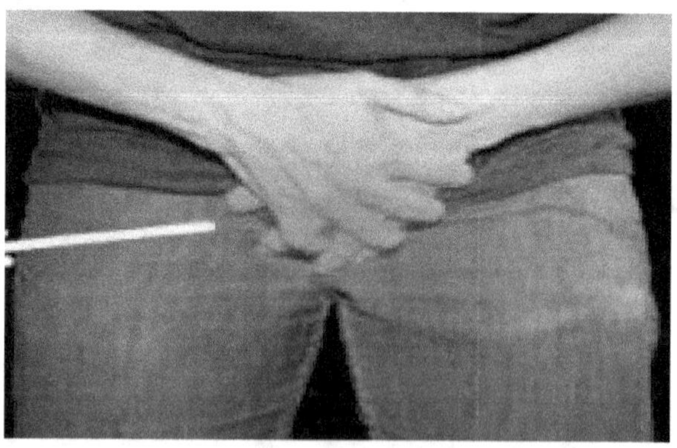

Gonorrhea Shows Early Symptoms in Men

Cervicitis

Cervicitis is inflammation of the cervix, often caused by infections such as chlamydia, gonorrhea, or herpes. Cervicitis is mostly a result of long-standing untreated sexually transmitted diseases. Most infections of gonorrhea and chlamydia are asymptomatic as a result of undiagnosed and untreated STIs. When this happens for too long the infection ascends into the cervix and uterus

When symptoms appeared, the symptoms may include abnormal vaginal discharge, vaginal bleeding (particularly after intercourse), pelvic pain, and dyspareunia. Cervicitis is differentiated from vaginal candidiasis based on the location of symptoms (cervix vs. vagina) and specific causative pathogens.

A thorough medical history, physical examination, laboratory testing, and diagnostic procedures may be necessary to establish an accurate diagnosis and determine the appropriate treatment plan.

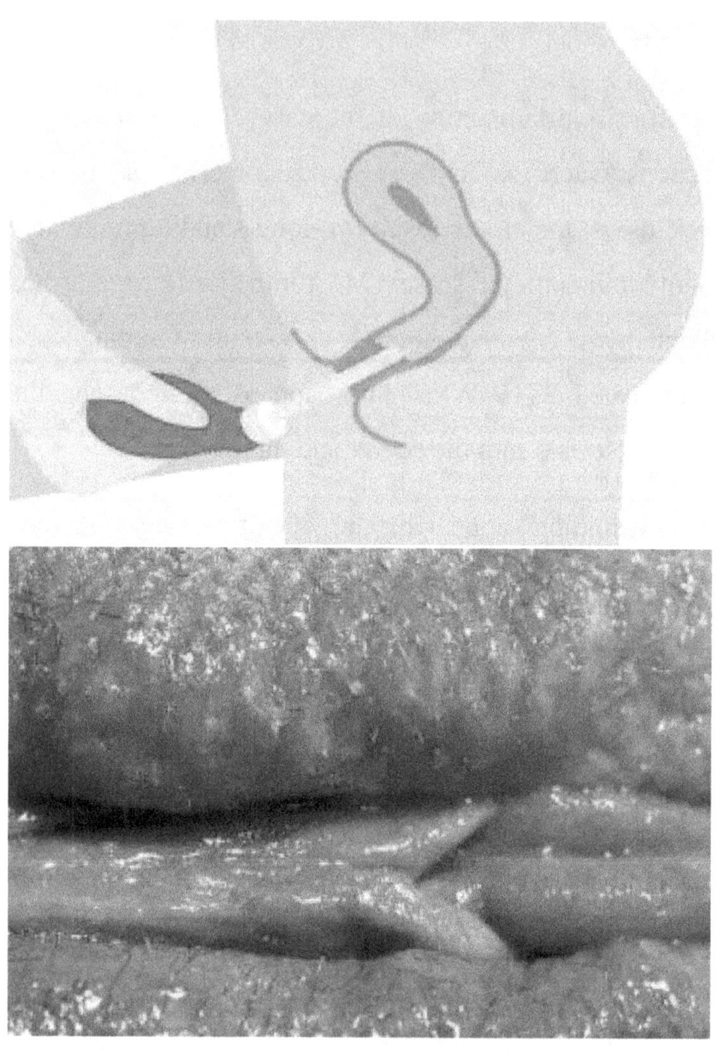

Risk factors and vaginal infections signs

CHAPTER 4

PREVENTION STRATEGIES

Prevention Strategies

Preventing vaginal candidiasis involves adopting strategies that help maintain a healthy vaginal environment and reduce the risk of Candida overgrowth. Most of the prevention strategies involve reversing or eliminating the risk factors. Some common preventive measures individuals can apply to prevent, control, or eliminate candidiasis infection are listed below.

Easily Modifiable Lifestyle Factors

Practice Good Genital Hygiene

Keep the genital area (only outside the vulva area) clean and dry by washing with mild, unscented soap and water daily, especially during menstruation. Change the menstrual pad frequently when soaked to keep the vagina dry. Avoid using harsh soaps, douches, feminine hygiene sprays, or scented products in the vaginal area, as they can disrupt the natural balance of vaginal flora and increase the risk of yeast infections, bacterial vaginosis, trichomonas vaginalis, and other genital tract infections.

Wear Breathable Underwear

Choose breathable, cotton underwear and avoid tight-fitting clothing that can trap moisture and heat in the genital area, creating an environment conducive to yeast growth. Change out of wet clothing, such as swimsuits or workout clothes, promptly after swimming or exercising. This helps to keep the vagina dry and prevent creating an enabling environment for candida growth.

Practice Safe Sex

Even though vaginal candidiasis or yeast infection is not a sexually transmitted infection, sex can increase the risk and recurrences of yeast infection in the vagina as explained above. Practicing safe sexual intercourse will therefore help to prevent, curtail, minimize, or control this infection. Use condoms consistently and correctly during sexual activity to reduce the risk of sexually transmitted infections (STIs) that can increase susceptibility to vaginal candidiasis. Limit the number of sexual partners and communicate openly with partners about symptoms of reproductive tract ill-health, especially STIs.

Avoid Unnecessary Antibiotic Use

Take antibiotics only when prescribed by a healthcare provider and follow the regimen carefully. Antibiotics can disrupt the balance of vaginal flora and increase the risk of yeast infections, so it's essential to use them judiciously and only when necessary. Most patients tend to extend medications, especially those that help alleviate their symptoms in the past.

Practice Aftercare for Vaginal Infections

If you have a history of recurrent yeast infections, talk to your physician about preventive measures or aftercare strategies, such as using over-the-counter antifungal treatments as directed or taking probiotics to help restore vaginal balance. This will help to balance the organisms in the vagina and prevent recurrences.

Regular Health Screenings

Attend regular gynecological check-ups and screenings to monitor vaginal health and detect any signs of infection early. Report any unusual vaginal symptoms to your healthcare provider promptly for evaluation and treatment.

Optimize Vaginal pH

Maintain a healthy vaginal pH by avoiding practices that can alter vaginal acidity, such as douching or using vaginal products containing harsh chemicals. Consuming a balanced diet rich in fruits, vegetables, and probiotic-rich foods may help promote vaginal health and maintain a healthy vaginal pH.

Managing Underlying Medical Conditions

Manage underlying medical conditions such as diabetes, HIV/AIDS, and immune disorders effectively to reduce the risk of recurrent yeast infections. Follow your doctor's recommendations for managing chronic conditions and maintaining optimal health. Most people with vaginal yeast do not however have any of the listed conditions as other factors predispose them than these.

Limit Sugary Foods and Beverages

Yeast thrives on sugar, so reducing your intake of sugary foods and beverages can be beneficial. Choose whole foods and limit processed foods, sweets, and sugary drinks.

Choose complex carbohydrates like whole grains (brown rice, quinoa, oats), legumes, and vegetables over refined carbohydrates (white bread, white rice, sugary cereals). Complex carbohydrates provide sustained energy and are less likely to spike blood sugar levels.

Eat healthy Fats including sources of healthy fats in your diet such as avocados, nuts, seeds, and fatty fish like salmon. These fats help support your immune system and reduce inflammation. Also, drink enough fluids to stay hydrated. Adequate hydration supports overall bodily functions, including maintaining healthy vaginal flora.

Avoid triggers of yeast infection in daily diet. Some individuals find that certain foods trigger yeast infections. Common triggers include alcohol, caffeine, and foods high in yeast or mold, such as bread and aged cheeses. Pay attention to your body and consider eliminating any foods that seem to exacerbate symptoms.

By incorporating these preventive strategies into your daily routine and lifestyle, you can help reduce the risk of developing vaginal candidiasis and maintain optimal vaginal health. Note that these measures are meant to prevent you from contracting the infection but once one is infected, treatment is required to control its progression and worsening to the next stage.

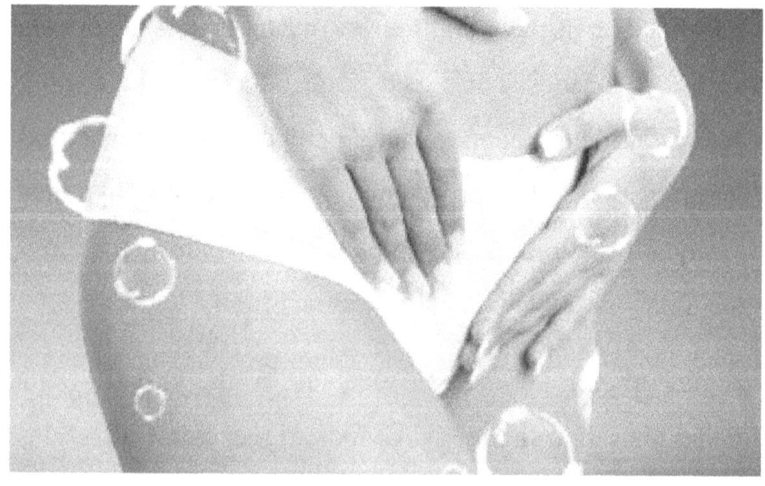

Neat Vagina Translate into Good Sex Life and Healthy Relationship

CHAPTER 5

MANAGEMENT OF YEAST INFECTION

There are different management options for vaginal candidiasis, depending on the severity and frequency of the infection, the type of Candida species involved, and the patient's preferences and medical conditions. This paper concentrates on vaginal candidiasis hence the treatment modalities are only explained for vaginal candidiasis.

The Azole Class of Medications

Azole: These drugs belong to the azole class of antifungals. They work by inhibiting the synthesis of ergosterol, a component of the fungal cell membrane. Azoles are effective against Candida albicans and some other Candida species but may have reduced activity against Candida glabrata and Candida krusei.

These are drugs that kill or stop the growth of fungi. They can be taken orally, applied topically, or inserted vaginally, depending on the product and the dosage. Antifungal medications are the first-line treatment for uncomplicated vaginal candidiasis, which is defined as a sporadic or infrequent infection, with mild to moderate symptoms, caused by Candida albicans. Some of the common antifungal medications used for vaginal candidiasis are clotrimazole, miconazole, butoconazole, terconazole, tioconazole, and fluconazole. Some of these exist over the counter.

Complicated vaginal candidiasis can be treated with antifungal medication, but may require longer or more intensive courses or alternative agents. For recurrent infections, defined as four or more episodes per year, the recommended treatment is a five to seven days course of oral fluconazole course followed by a once-weekly fluconazole maintenance regimen for six months. For severe infections, defined as extensive vulvar erythema, edema, excoriation, or fissure formation, the recommended treatment is a short course of oral fluconazole, plus a topical antifungal agent for symptom relief.

Itraconazole: Itraconazole is an oral antifungal medication that may be used to treat vaginal candidiasis. It works similarly to fluconazole by inhibiting fungal growth. It is less commonly prescribed for this purpose compared to fluconazole which is far safer and tolerable.

Ketoconazole: Ketoconazole is an antifungal medication that may be used orally to treat vaginal yeast infections, although it is less commonly prescribed for this purpose due to the availability of other more effective options. Ketoconazole interferes with the synthesis of ergosterol, a crucial component of fungal cell membranes.

Treatment of Non-albicans or Recurrent Candidiasis

For non-albicans candidiasis, which may be resistant to fluconazole, the recommended treatment is a topical antifungal agent, such as clotrimazole, miconazole, or butoconazole, or an alternative oral agent, such as itraconazole or voriconazole. For women with diabetes, immunosuppression, or other underlying conditions, the recommended treatment is the same as for uncomplicated infections. They may need closer follow-up and monitoring for possible complications or recurrence of side effects.

The Role of Topical Antifungals

They are applied directly to the affected area, such as the skin, mouth, or vagina. They include creams, ointments, suppositories, tablets, or lozenges that contain antifungal agents such as clotrimazole, miconazole, nystatin, butoconazole, or terconazole. Topical antifungals are effective against most Candida species. They are usually used for mild to moderate cases of cutaneous, oral, or vaginal candidiasis, or as an adjunct to oral or intravenous therapy.

The Role Vaginal Pessaries for Candidiasis Treatment

Some azoles can be given in a form of a capsule that is inserted in the vagina for about 3 to 7 days. These are sometimes used in the management of yeast infections, particularly in cases of recurrent or resistant infections. They are typical antifungal agents such as clotrimazole, miconazole, or nystatin.

Vaginal pessaries deliver medication directly to the site of infection, providing targeted treatment to the affected area and allowing for a higher concentration of antifungal medication to be delivered directly to the vagina compared to oral medications, potentially increasing effectiveness. The good thing is that most pessaries are combined with other medications making them effective against other infections such as trichomoniasis and bacterial vaginosis as these infections mostly co-exist. They are often convenient to use and can be inserted at home without needing a healthcare provider's assistance.

There may be fewer systemic side effects than oral antifungal medications because the pessaries are applied locally. In cases of recurrent yeast infections, using vaginal pessaries as a maintenance treatment may help prevent future episodes by keeping the yeast population in check. vaginal pessaries offer an alternative treatment option. Vaginal pessaries also offer an alternative treatment option for individuals who do not respond well to oral antifungal medications or have contraindications to them.

They can also be used with other treatments such as oral antifungal medications or topical creams for more severe or persistent infections.

It's important to note that while vaginal pessaries can be effective for many women with yeast infections, they may not be suitable for everyone. Some patients feel some inconvenience in inserting these medicated capsules into the vagina. Adolescent virgins or celibacy may also not be able to insert pessaries deep into the vagina due to interference of the hymen. Most healthcare professionals therefore avoid prescribing pessaries to virgins due to their shyness, inability to insert, and the possibility of breaking the vaginal hymen with insertable pessaries.

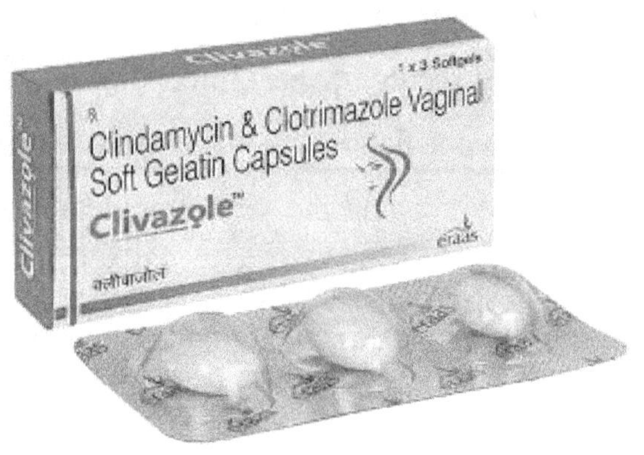

Combined antifungal pessaries

Echinocandins class of medications

Echinocandins: A class of antifungals that includes caspofungin, micafungin, and anidulafungin. They work by inhibiting the synthesis of beta-glucan, a component of the fungal cell wall. Echinocandins are effective against most Candida species. Echinocandins are given intravenously for invasive candidiasis and are not used for yeast infection treatment. They can cause side effects such as infusion reactions, rash, or liver problems.

Amphotericin B: An intravenous medication that belongs to the polyene class of antifungals. It works by binding to ergosterol and creating pores in the fungal cell membrane. Amphotericin B is effective against most of the candida species that cause vaginal yeast infection. Amphotericin B is usually reserved for severe or refractory cases of invasive candidiasis, or for patients who cannot tolerate other antifungals. Amphotericin B can cause side effects.

The Role of Probiotics in Candidiasis Treatment

Probiotics are live microorganisms that can have beneficial effects on the health of the host. They are often found in fermented foods, such as yogurt, or in dietary supplements. Probiotics can help maintain the balance of bacteria and yeast in the vagina, which is important for preventing and treating vaginal candidiasis.

Probiotics work by competing with Candida for nutrients and space in the vagina, and inhibiting its growth and adhesion to the vaginal cells. It also produces substances, such as lactic acid, hydrogen peroxide, and bacteriocins, that lower the pH of the vagina and create an unfavorable environment for Candida. It enhances the immune system and the mucosal barrier of the vagina and modulates the inflammatory response to Candida.

Therefore, more research is needed to determine the optimal use of probiotics for vaginal candidiasis. By writing this book, I do not personally recommend the use of probiotics for vaginal yeast infections. If you are interested in trying probiotics for this condition, you should consult your healthcare provider first in your state for recommendations. You should also follow the instructions on the product label and monitor for any side effects or adverse reactions.

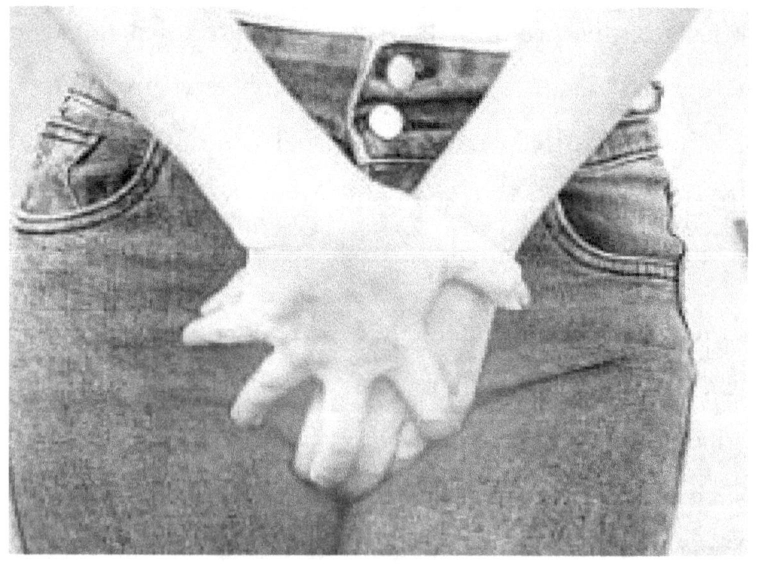

There is severe intense itching in vaginal candidiasis

Prescription for Uncomplicated Vulvovaginal candidiasis

- ✓ Tab Fluconazole 150mg stat
- ✓ Clotrimazole cream

Prescription for Uncomplicated Vulvovaginal candidiasis for virgins and celibacy who cannot insert pessaries

- ✓ Tab Fluconazole 150mg stat

Prescription for severe Vulvovaginal candidiasis

- ✓ Tab Fluconazole 150mg stat
- ✓ Clotrimazole vaginal pessaries 200mg nocte for 3days

OR

- ✓ Tab Fluconazole 150mg stat
- ✓ Miconazole vaginal pessaries 400mg nocte for 3 days
- ✓ Miconazole or clotrimazole cream

Prescription for severe Vulvovaginal Candidiasis for Celibacy

- ✓ Tab Fluconazole 150mg daily for 5ays
- ✓ Clotrimazole or miconazole cream to apply

Prescription for Mix Vulvovaginitis

- ✓ Tab Fluconazole 150mg stat
- ✓ Clotrimazole+ Clindamycin Vaginal Pessaries 1 Tablet Nocte for 3 Days
- ✓ Clotrimazole cream

Prescription for Recurrent Vulvovaginal candidiasis

- ✓ Tab Fluconazole 150mg daily for 7 days, and 150mg once weekly for 6 months

Note: The cream helps to reduce the burning sensation and itching of the vulvar. Some pharmaceutical companies produced a combination drug with hydrocortisone. The hydrocortisone component offers fast relief from intense itching and burning sensation whilst the antifungal medications inhibit the growth of yeast.

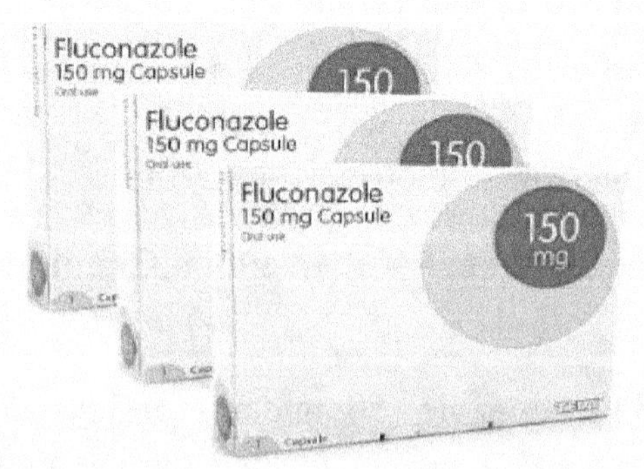

Fluconazole for Curing Yeast Infection

Inserting cloves and garlic can cure vaginal yeast infections: I have encountered a good number of clients who insert various substances into the vagina for numerous reasons. Some people believe that inserting garlic cloves into the vagina can help treat vaginal itching caused by yeast infections. There is however no scientific evidence to support this claim. This practice can be harmful as it introduces foreign organisms into the vagina leading to vulva irritation and infection. It does not enhance reproductive health.

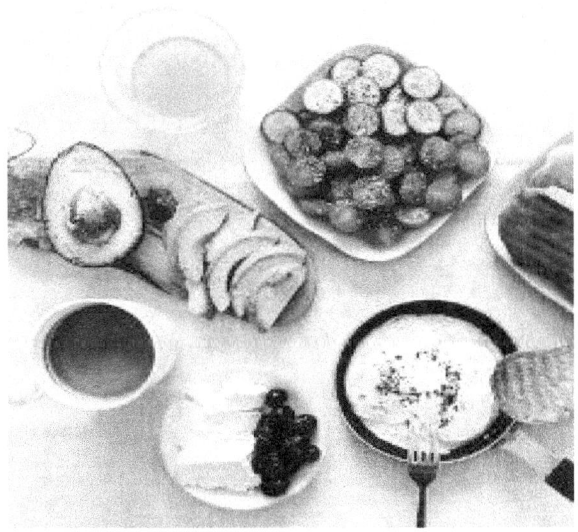

Inserting Food in the Vagina is Unrecommended

Vaginal itch creams can treat yeast infections: These products may provide temporary relief for the itching, irritation, and burning sensation during urination, but they do not address the underlying cause of the infection. To treat and prevent recurrent yeast infections, you need to use an antifungal medication that kills the excess yeast.

Yeast infections are sexually transmitted: Yeast infections affect the reproductive tract in both men and women and on very rare occasions can be passed to sexual partners. They are however not classified as sexually transmitted infections (STIs). Celibacy or virgins do get vaginal yeast infections. Vaginal yeast infections are caused by an imbalance of the normal flora in the vagina by lifestyle changes in individuals.

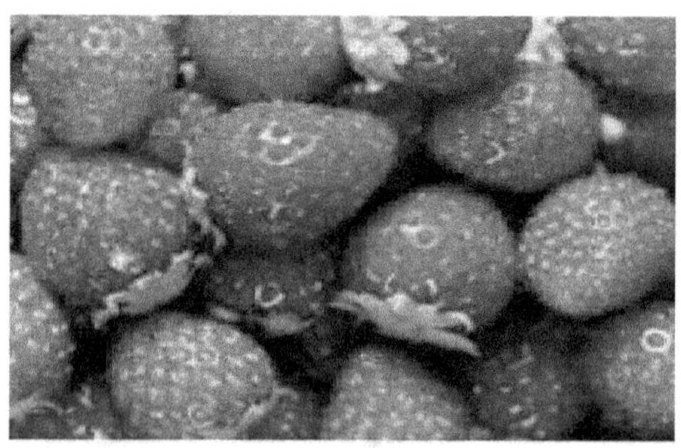

Common Foods Mostly Inserted in the Vagina

CHAPTER 6

CONCLUSION

Candidiasis is a fungal infection caused by the overgrowth of Candida species, commonly Candida albicans, which naturally inhabit various parts of the human body, including the skin, mouth, throat, gut, and genital tract. Infection of the vagina is known as vaginal yeast infections or vaginal candidiasis or vulvovaginal candidiasis.

The symptoms of vaginal candidiasis include cheese-like vaginal discharge, vulvar itching, burning sensation, and redness or vulvar swelling.

Antifungal creams, ointments, or suppositories are available over-the-counter (OTC) at pharmacies and drugstores for vaginal candidiasis treatment. Common OTC antifungal medications for vaginal candidiasis include clotrimazole cream or pessaries, miconazole cream or pessaries, tioconazole, and 150mg of fluconazole.

These products are typically applied intravaginally for 1 to 7 days, depending on the product and formulation.

It's essential to follow the instructions provided with the medication carefully and complete the full course of treatment, even if symptoms improve before finishing.

In some cases, combination therapy, which involves using both oral and intravaginal antifungal medications simultaneously for more effective treatment of severe or recurrent vaginal candidiasis.

Some individuals may choose to use alternative or complementary therapies for the treatment of vaginal candidiasis, although evidence supporting their effectiveness is limited. These therapies may include probiotics, herbal remedies, or dietary supplements. It's essential to avoid alternative therapies, as they may interact with other medications or conditions.

Lifestyle modifications such as practicing good genital hygiene, wearing breathable underwear, practicing safe sex, avoiding unnecessary antibiotic use, optimizing vaginal pH, limiting sugary foods and beverages, and regular health screenings are important to prevent yeast infections.

WISH YOU GOOD VAGINAL HEALTH